Guard Your Glow

A Smart Girl's Guide to Period Confidence

Eunice C. Mingo, LPC-S

The Efficient Coach

ISBN: 979-8-9957573-0-6

Printed in the United States of America.

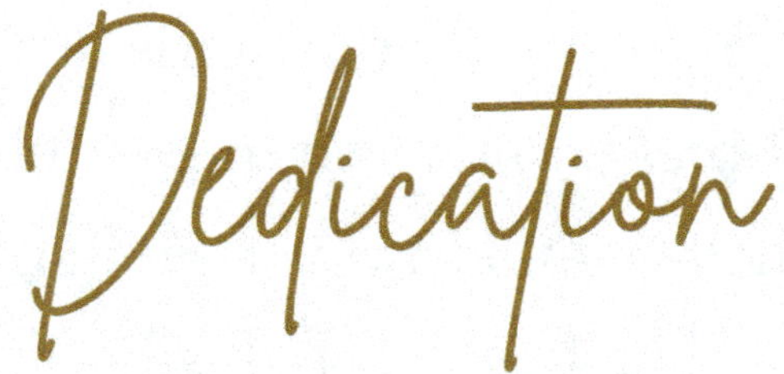

To every girl learning her rhythm,
May you grow without shame,
Rest without guilt,
And become who God created you to be
unapologetically.

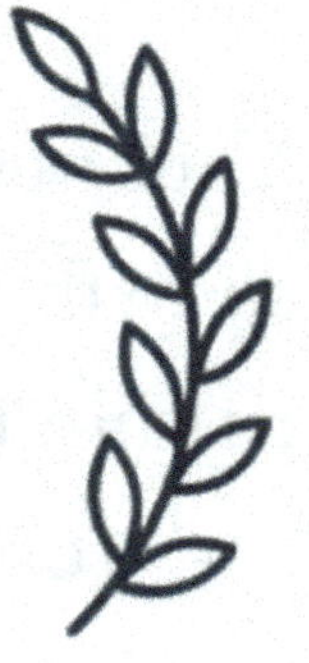

~ Eunice

The Efficient Coach

Welcome to a No-Shame Space

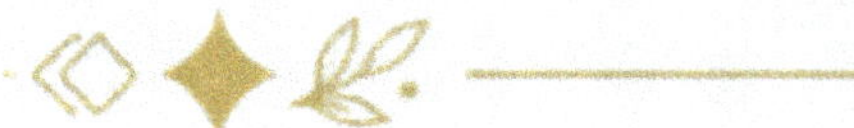

Your body is changing on purpose. Some girls learn about their periods in calm conversations at home. Some learn in health class. Some quietly search for answers on their own. However, you arrived here, you are not behind. You are growing. The beauty of this book is that it speaks clearly and does not whisper.

Your period is not something that suddenly happened to you. It is something your body prepared for long before you noticed. It is part of a rhythm that connects you to women and girls who came before you.

- You deserve to understand your body.
- You deserve confidence.
- You deserve peace.

Affirmation

I am learning my body with courage and confidence.

This book provides educational and emotional wellness guidance.
It is not a substitute for medical care. Always speak with a trusted adult or healthcare provider for specific concerns.

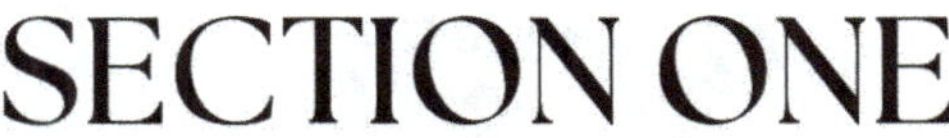

SECTION ONE

Glow Roots

Understanding your value is where confidence begins.

Girl, You Better Glow:

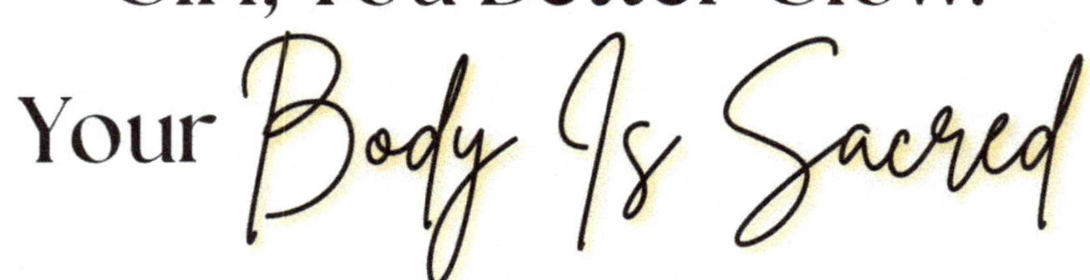

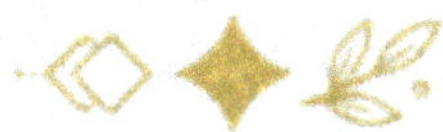

Before we talk about periods, products, or patterns, we begin with something more important: **Value.**

Your body is sacred.
Sacred means deeply valuable and worthy of respect. It does not mean perfect. There is no such thing as perfect. Sacred means important. It means something is worthy of care, attention, and protection. Your body is not random, nor is it accident. It is wonderfully designed. It does a lot without you even having to ask. For example, your body breathes while you sleep. It heals your cuts. It digests your food. It balances hormones. It grows, strengthens, and repairs itself every single day of your life. Even when you are not paying attention, your body is working on your behalf.

Your menstrual cycle is one of those powerful systems. When your period begins, it is not your body turning against you. It is your body stepping into a new level of growth. It is part of a rhythm that has been quietly preparing inside you for years.

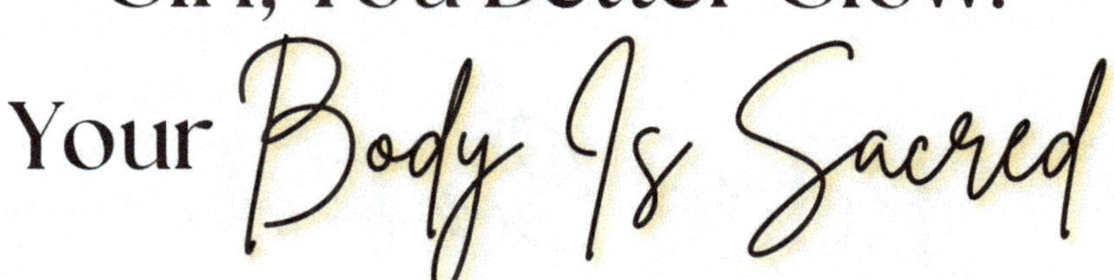

Girl, You Better Glow: Your Body Is Sacred

Across many African cultures and throughout the African diaspora, a girl's first menstrual cycle has long been recognized as an important transition. It was acknowledged with guidance, wisdom, and care. Elder women gathered with girls to teach them about dignity, responsibility, and self-respect. They created space for learning and preparation. These traditions were rooted in education, protection, and community. Cultural traditions differ across families and communities, and each family may choose to recognize growth in its own way. **This history matters. Our history will always matter.**

Long before advertisements told women to whisper about their cycles, many communities understood menstruation as strength, continuity, and preparation for adulthood. You stand in that lineage. Your body is not something to hide. It is something to understand. It is something to honor with wisdom and care. Guarding your glow begins with knowing your worth.

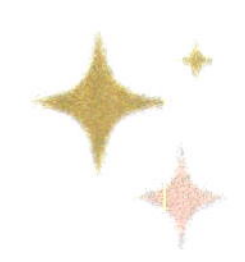

Edge *Control*

Edge control means protecting your peace before your feelings take over. It means pausing, breathing, and responding with confidence instead of reacting in confusion.

You are not behind.
You are not weird.
You are not alone.

You are growing.
Growth is and always will be sacred.

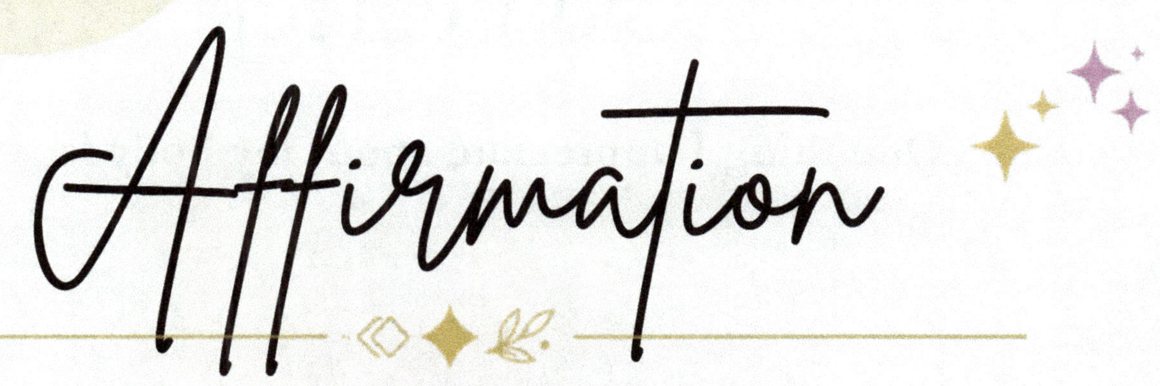

My body is sacred.

I treat it with respect and care.

I honor my growth with confidence.

Glow Check

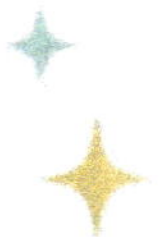

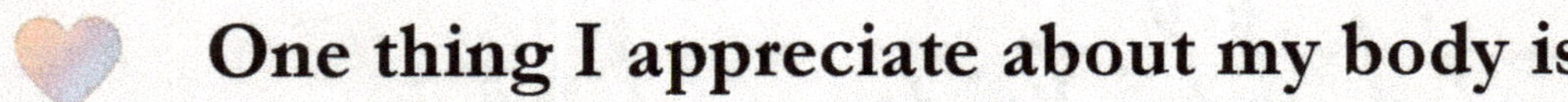

One thing I appreciate about my body is

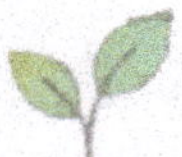

When I think about growth, I feel

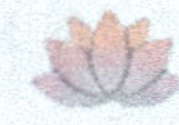

I can honor my body by

Sacred and Growing

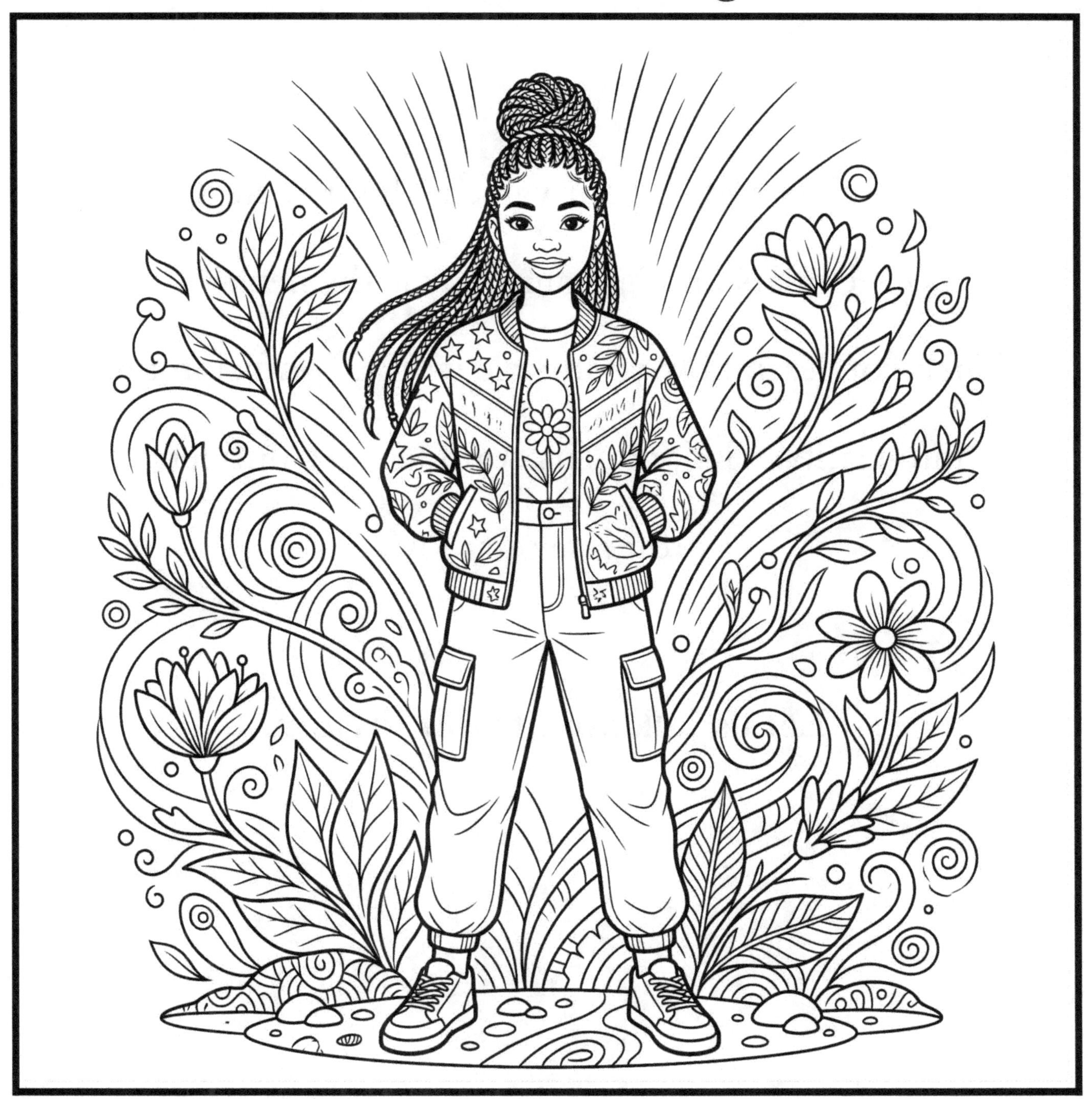

Color slowly and think about one thing you are proud of.

Understanding your value is the first step.

Understanding your body is the next.

When you learn how your cycle works, confusion turns into clarity. Clarity builds confidence. Confidence protects your glow.

Let us talk about your rhythm.

SECTION TWO

Your Rhythm. Your Rules.

Understanding your value is where confidence begins.

What a Period Is

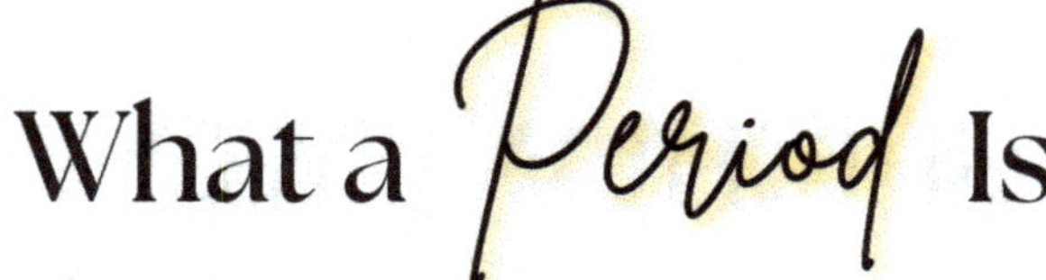

A period happens when the lining inside your uterus sheds and leaves your body through the vagina. Each month, your body builds this lining in preparation for the possibility of pregnancy in the future. When pregnancy does not occur, the lining releases. This is not dirt leaving your body. It is not punishment or a mistake. It is biology.

Your period may last between three and seven days. In the first few years, your cycle may not arrive at the same time each month. That is normal but always keep the beginning date and the ending of your cycle in your calendar. During this time of the month, your hormones are learning to coordinate.

What a Period Is

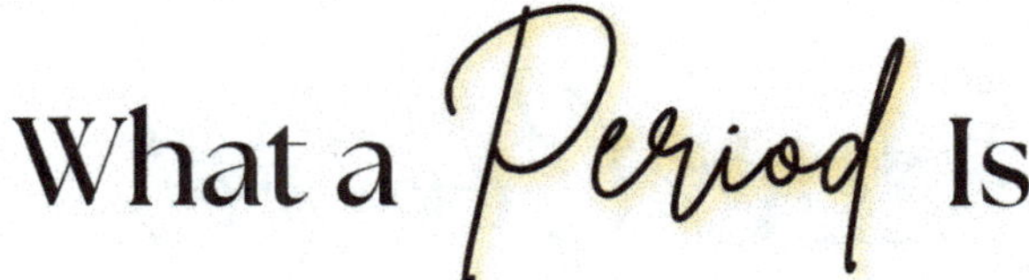

Hormones are chemical messengers that travel through your bloodstream. They tell different systems in your body what to do. Estrogen and progesterone help regulate your menstrual cycle. They can influence your mood, your sleep, your energy, and even your ability to concentrate. Understanding what is happening inside your body replaces fear with knowledge. When you understand your cycle, you feel less surprised and more prepared.

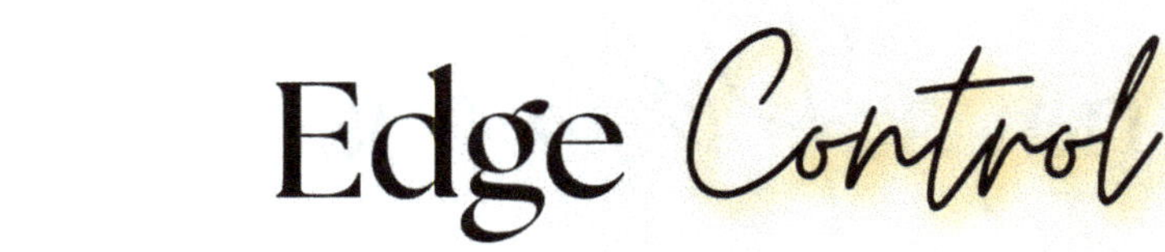

Edge *Control*

**When something feels new,
it can feel overwhelming.**

Instead of worrying about what you may not understand, pause and remind yourself that your body knows what it is doing.

Clarity helps your emotions move to a calm space. Your body is learning and so are you.

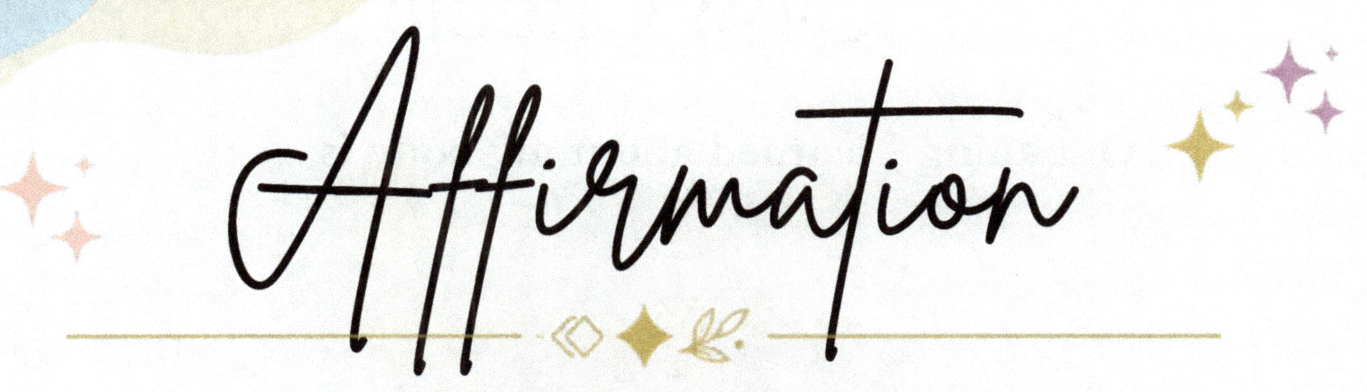

My cycle is natural, and my body knows what it is doing. I move with understanding instead of fear.

Glow Check

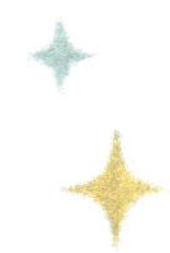

One thing I learned about my body is

Knowing this makes me feel

When I understand something new, I

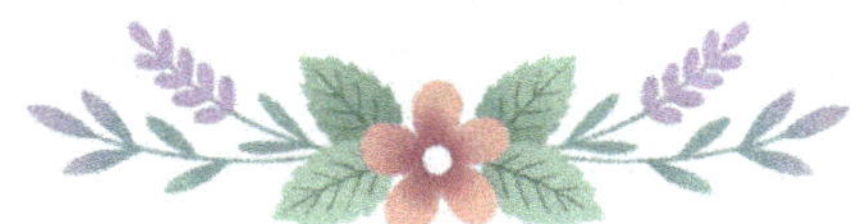

Trust the Rhythm

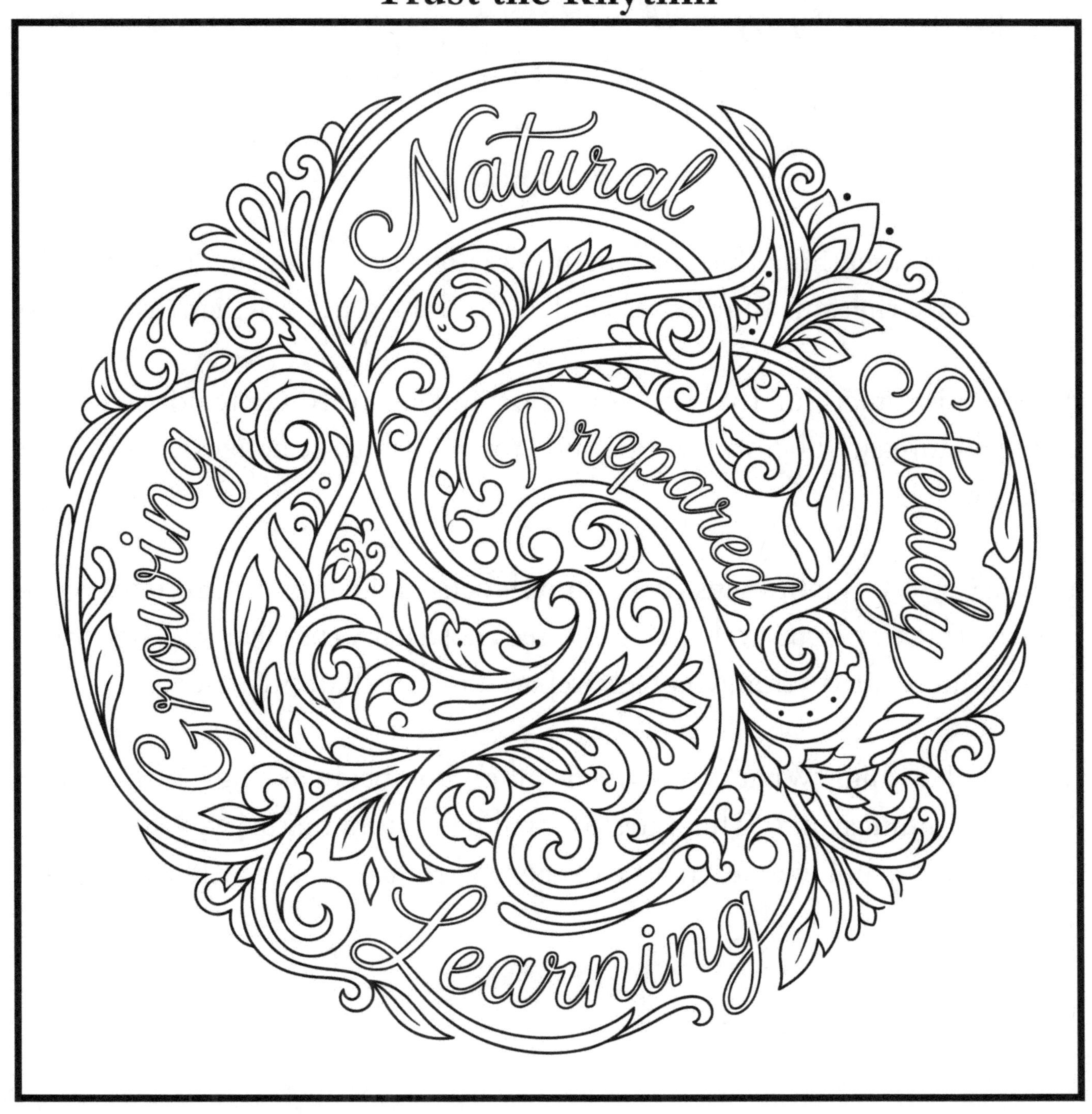

Rhythm and Patterns

A *rhythm* is something that repeats in a steady way. Music has rhythm. The seasons have rhythm. Your heartbeat has rhythm. Your cycle has rhythm too.

A *pattern* is something that happens again and again. You may notice that you feel more tired before your period. You may notice changes in your appetite.

You may also feel more sensitive or more focused during certain times of the month. Tracking your cycle helps you see those patterns clearly. When you understand your rhythm, you feel prepared rather than surprised.

Instead of asking, "What is wrong with me?" you begin asking, "What is my body communicating?" That question will help build maturity. When you learn your rhythm, you learn how to move with it instead of fighting against it.

That is definitely a superpower.

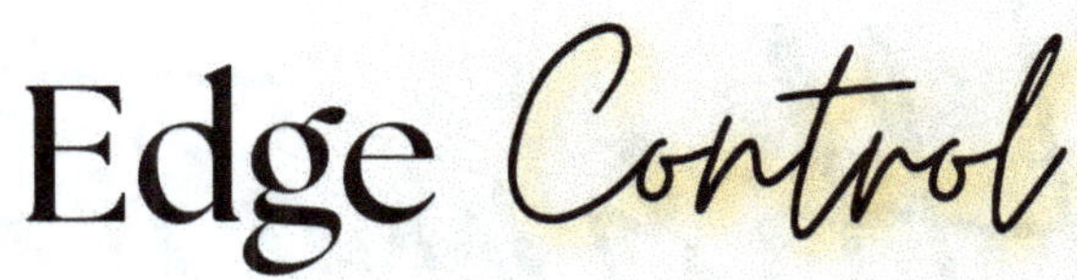

Edge Control

Instead of reacting to everything I feel,
I will pause and observe.

Ask yourself what your body may need.
Awareness is a form of protection.

You are learning to guard your glow
with wisdom.

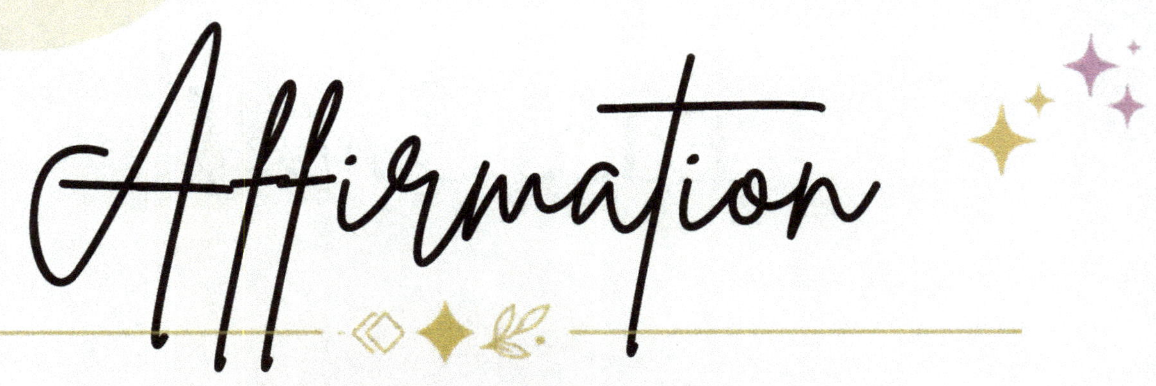

I learn my rhythm

so I can move with confidence.

I listen to my body with respect.

Glow Check

A pattern I have noticed is

When I track my cycle, I feel

Listening to my body helps me

My Rhythm Tracker

MONTH:________________ YEAR:________________

MON	TUE	WED	THU	FRI	SAT	SUN

GOALS & DREAMS	
NOTES & DOODLES	

Your rhythm belongs to you.

Cycle & Habit Tracker

MONTH ____________________ **YEAR** ____________________

MOOD     

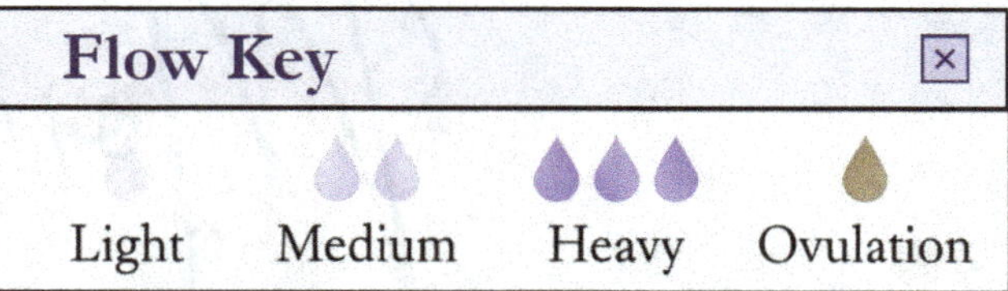

DAYS	1	2	3	4	5	6	7	8	9	10	11	12	13	14	15	16	17	18	19	20	21	22	23	24	25	26	27	28	29	30	31
CYCLE FLOW (Color In)	○	○	○	○	○	○	○	○	○	○	○	○	○	○	○	○	○	○	○	○	○	○	○	○	○	○	○	○	○	○	○
DRANK 8 GLASSES OF WATER	○	○	○	○	○	○	○	○	○	○	○	○	○	○	○	○	○	○	○	○	○	○	○	○	○	○	○	○	○	○	○
EXERCISE (30 MINS)	○	○	○	○	○	○	○	○	○	○	○	○	○	○	○	○	○	○	○	○	○	○	○	○	○	○	○	○	○	○	○
READ FOR 15 MINS	○	○	○	○	○	○	○	○	○	○	○	○	○	○	○	○	○	○	○	○	○	○	○	○	○	○	○	○	○	○	○
SCINCARE ROUTINE	○	○	○	○	○	○	○	○	○	○	○	○	○	○	○	○	○	○	○	○	○	○	○	○	○	○	○	○	○	○	○
SLEEP (8 HOURS)	○	○	○	○	○	○	○	○	○	○	○	○	○	○	○	○	○	○	○	○	○	○	○	○	○	○	○	○	○	○	○

SECTION THREE

Move Boldly

You do not have to shrink because you are growing.

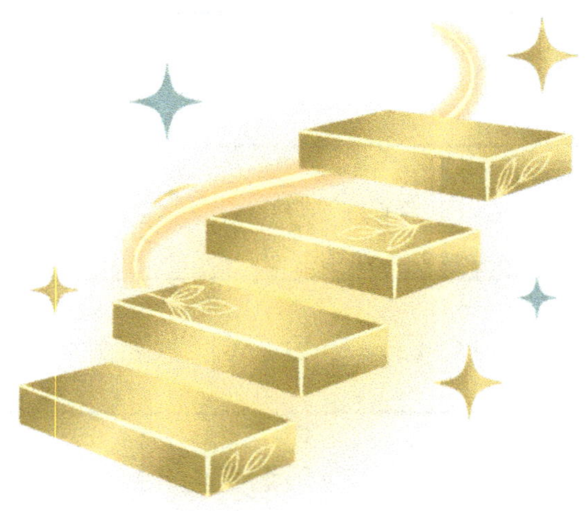

"You may encounter many defeats,
but you must not be defeated."
— *Maya Angelou*

If you are a dancer, gymnast, runner, cheerleader, basketball player, soccer player, or athlete of any kind, your body is already disciplined and powerful. You stretch it. You strengthen it. You trust it to perform. Your menstrual cycle works alongside that effort. Some days you may feel flexible and energized. Your jumps may feel lighter. Your turn may feel sharp. Your stride may feel strong. Other days you may feel heavier or more sensitive. Your lower back might ache. Your stomach might feel tight. You may feel more tired than usual.

That does not mean you are weak or strange. It means your body is balancing the energy it has. When you move frequently, your body sweats more. Sweat is your body's natural cooling system. During your period, when you are also sweating, you may notice more moisture. That is normal. Your body is working hard, and it is doing exactly what it was designed to do.

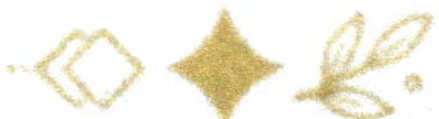

Because you are perspiring more, you may need to change your pad, tampon, or menstrual cup more often. That is not a problem. That is preparation. Preparation builds peace.

If you know you have practice or a game, pack a small period kit in your dance bag or sports bag. Include:

- **Extra pads, tampons, or cup supplies**
- **An extra pair of underwear**
- **Extra tights or shorts if needed**
- **Wipes or disposable washcloths**
- **A small plastic bag for used items**

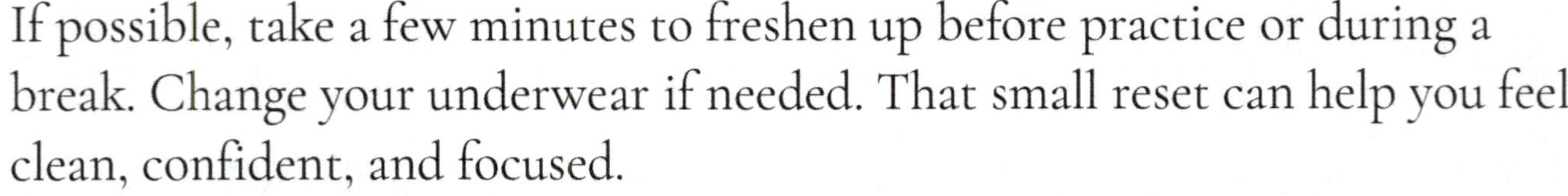

If possible, take a few minutes to freshen up before practice or during a break. Change your underwear if needed. That small reset can help you feel clean, confident, and focused.

Layer during practice if that makes you feel secure. Stay hydrated. Drink water. Fuel your body with nourishing foods. Your muscles and your cycle both require energy.

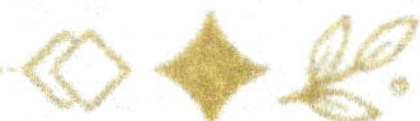

Move fully.

Extend your arms. Leap. Turn. Run. Take up space. You do not have to shrink because you are bleeding.

You do not have to sit out unless your body truly needs rest. Listening to your body is strength in action.

Some athletes notice that their performance shifts during different parts of their cycle. That information is valuable. When you learn your rhythm, you can plan accordingly.

You can prepare intentionally. You can work with your body instead of fighting against it. Resilience is already within you. Your ability to recover, adjust, and continue moving forward is part of who you are.

Guard your edges. Protect your peace. Shine with steady confidence.

Edge Control

**When your body feels different,
pause instead of panicking.**

**Notice what you need.
Adjust with calm confidence.**

**Strength is not about ignoring your body.
Strength is about honoring it.**

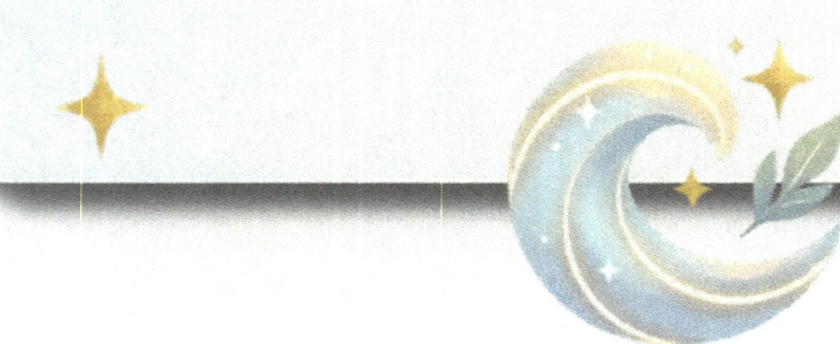

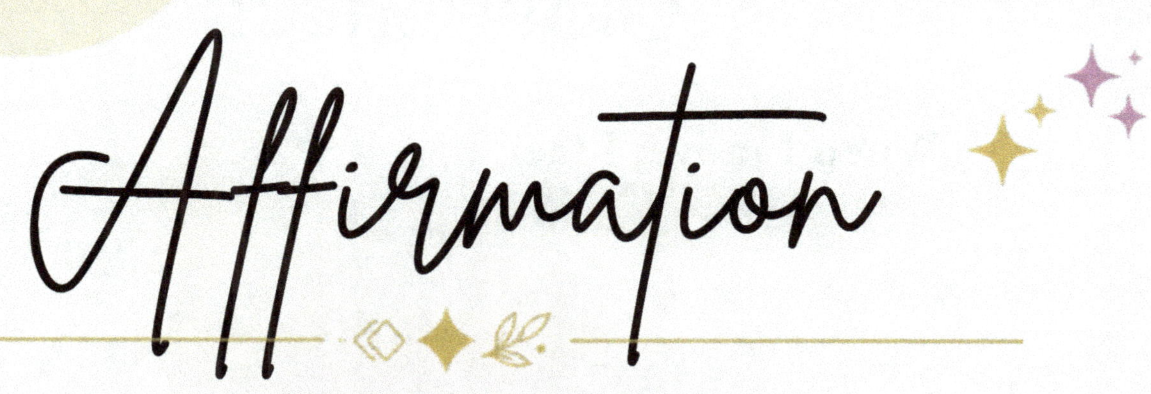

I move with awareness,

grace, and confidence.

My body is strong. I am resilient.

Glow Check

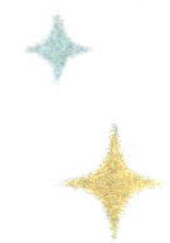

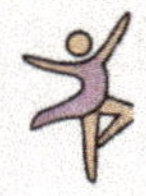

When I move, I feel

One way I can prepare for practice is

Listening to my body helps me

Strong. Steady. Resilient.

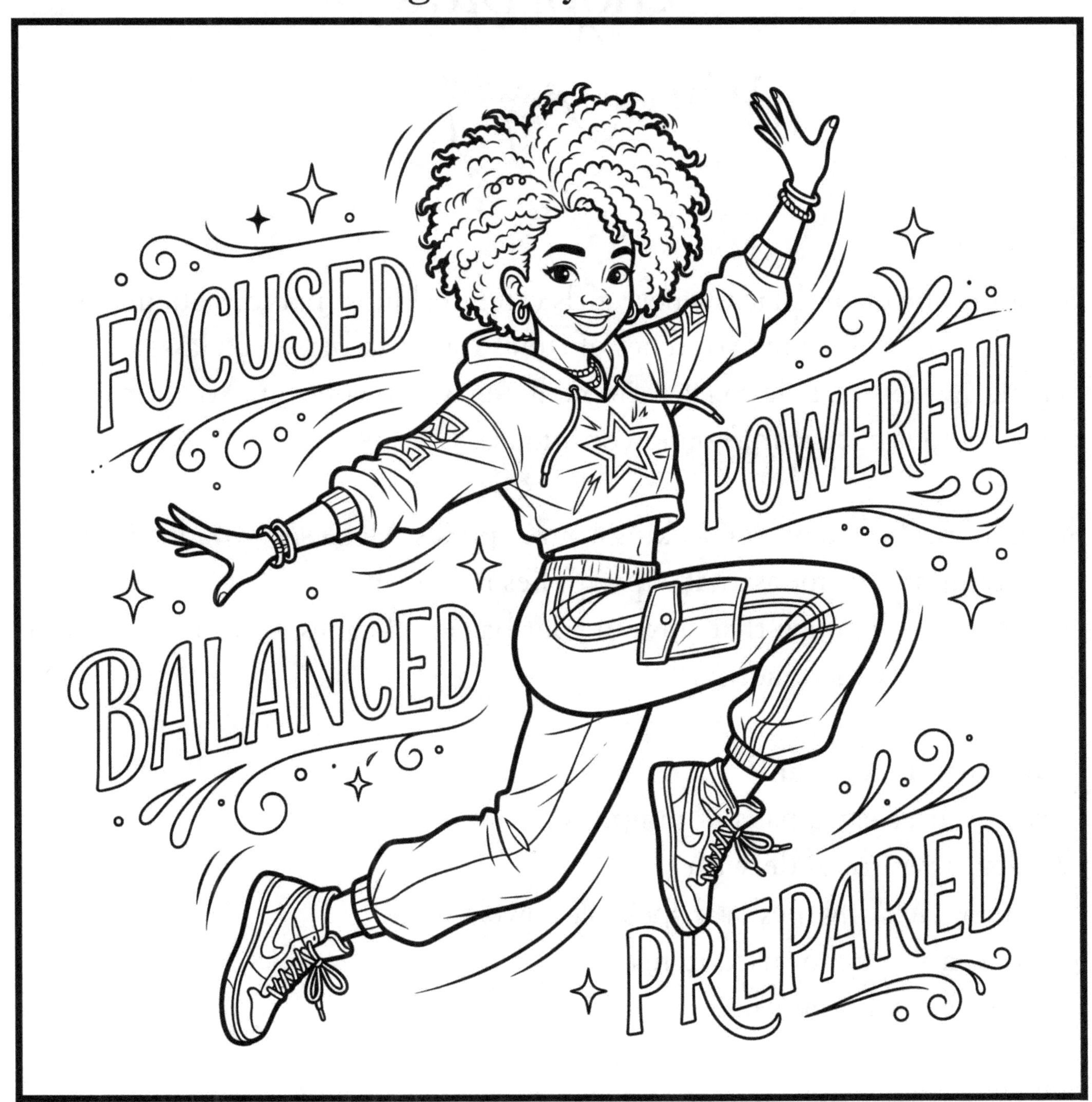

School Days With *Confidence*

School is one of the places where girls often feel most nervous about their periods. You sit for long stretches of time. You walk between classes. You may not always be able to leave immediately when you want to. Preparation turns nervous energy into quiet confidence.

Start your school day by checking your supplies. Make sure you have enough pads, tampons, or menstrual cup supplies in your backpack. Consider keeping a small pouch that stays in your bag at all times, so you do not have to remember it each month.

Your pouch may include:

- Two to three extra pads or tampons
- An extra pair of underwear
- A small pack of wipes or disposable towels
- A resealable bag for used items
- Travel-size hand sanitizer

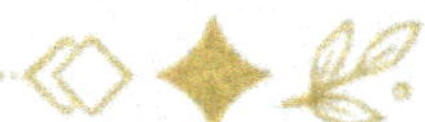

If your flow is heavier on certain days, plan to change your pad or tampon every few hours. Setting a quiet reminder can help you stay on schedule. When you need to ask a teacher to use the restroom, keep it simple. You can say, "May I please use the restroom?" That is enough.
If a teacher says no and you truly need to go, advocate calmly. You can say, "It is important." Most adults understand more than you think.

Make sure you choose clothing that makes you feel secure. Some girls prefer darker bottoms on heavier days. Others prefer shorts under skirts for extra protection. These choices are about comfort, not fear.
Millions of girls attend school during their periods every single day, so you are not alone.

Your period does not make you less intelligent.
It does not make you less capable.
It does not make you less confident.
It is simply one part of your growing body.

When you prepare, your mind is free to focus on learning, laughing, and being present with your friends.

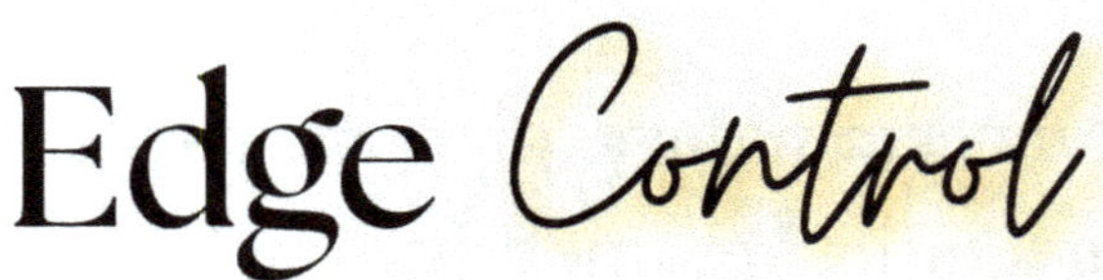

Edge Control

If you feel nervous at school, pause and breathe before letting worry take over.

Preparation is protection.

Calm is power.

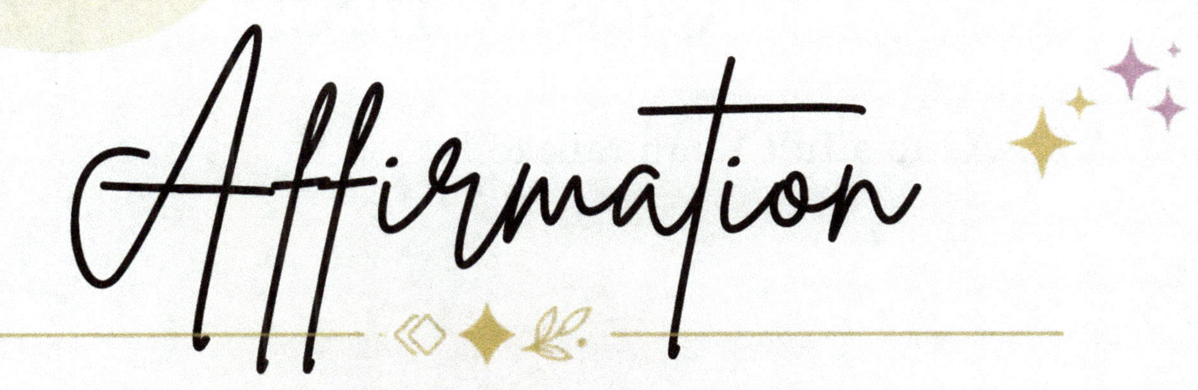

I am prepared.

I am capable.

I can handle any day with calm confidence.

Glow Check

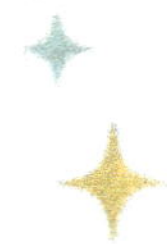

 **One adult I can talk to is**

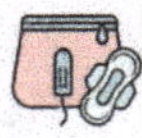 **My period pouch will include**

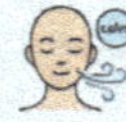 **When I feel nervous, I can**

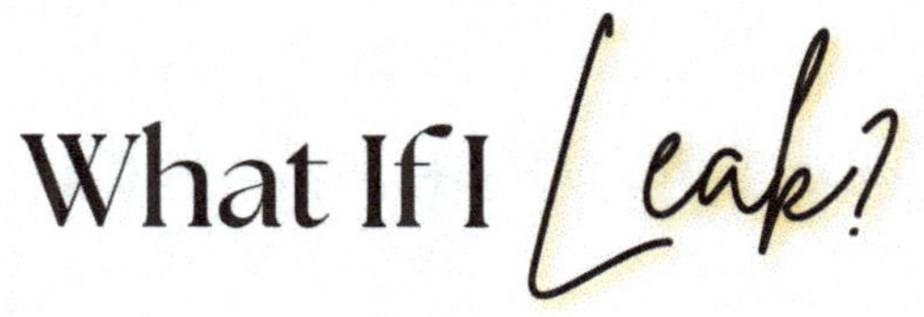

What If I Leak?

Almost every girl worries about this at some point.

You may wonder what would happen if someone notices. You may worry about standing up and seeing a stain. You may feel nervous about light-colored clothing or sitting for too long.

Take a slow breath.

Leaking can happen. It does not mean you did something wrong. It does not mean you did something wrong. It does not mean you were careless. It simply means your flow was heavier than expected or your product needed changing. That is not embarrassing. It is biology. Your body is still learning its rhythm. In the first few years, your cycle may not be predictable. Some days will be light. Some days will be heavier. Some months may surprise you. Surprises do not equal shame.

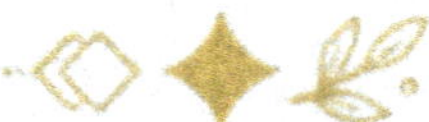

If you notice a leak, stay steady. Tie a sweatshirt or jacket around your waist if needed. Ask to use the restroom. Clean up and change your pad, tampon, or underwear. Reach out to a trusted adult if you need support. Most of the time, others notice far less than we imagine. If someone does notice, their reaction reflects their maturity, not your worth.

Even grown women have leak stories. It is a shared experience, even if people do not talk about it often. Confidence is not about never leaking. Confidence is knowing you can handle unexpected moments calmly.
Each time you are prepared, that helps. Always carry extra supplies. Know where restrooms are located. Trust that you can manage what happens.

A leak does not erase your glow.

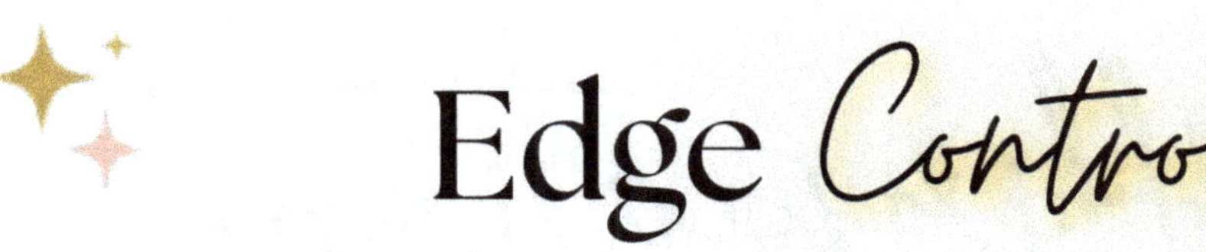

Edge Control

Pause. Breathe in slowly.
Hold. Breathe out gently.

Tell yourself, "I am okay. I can handle this."

Taking a pause to calm yourself
protects your confidence.

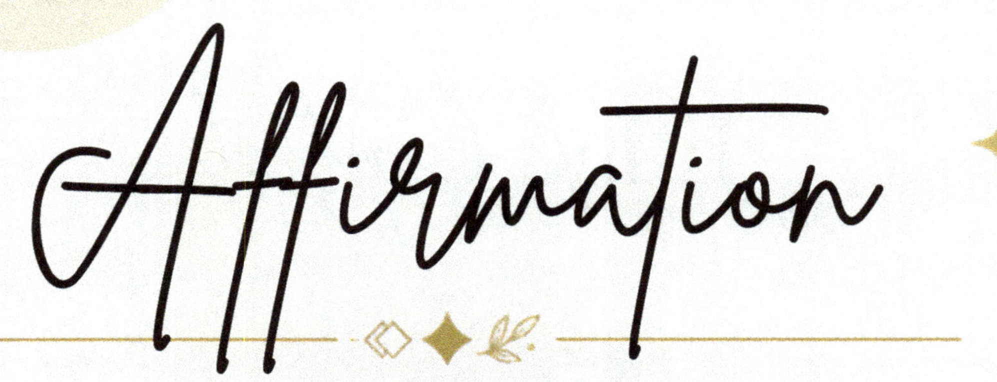

I can handle unexpected moments.

I stay calm and steady.

My glow is not erased by accidents.

Glow Check

If something unexpected happens, I can

A calming phrase I like is

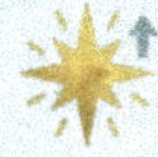

I know that I am still

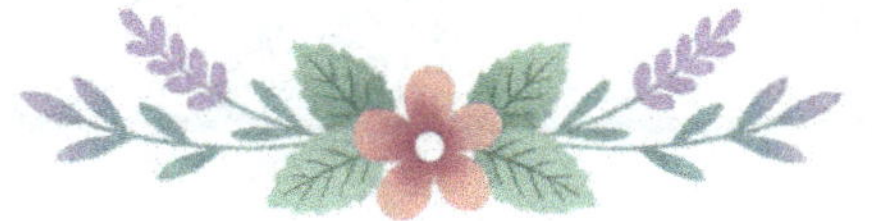

Accidents Do Not Define Me

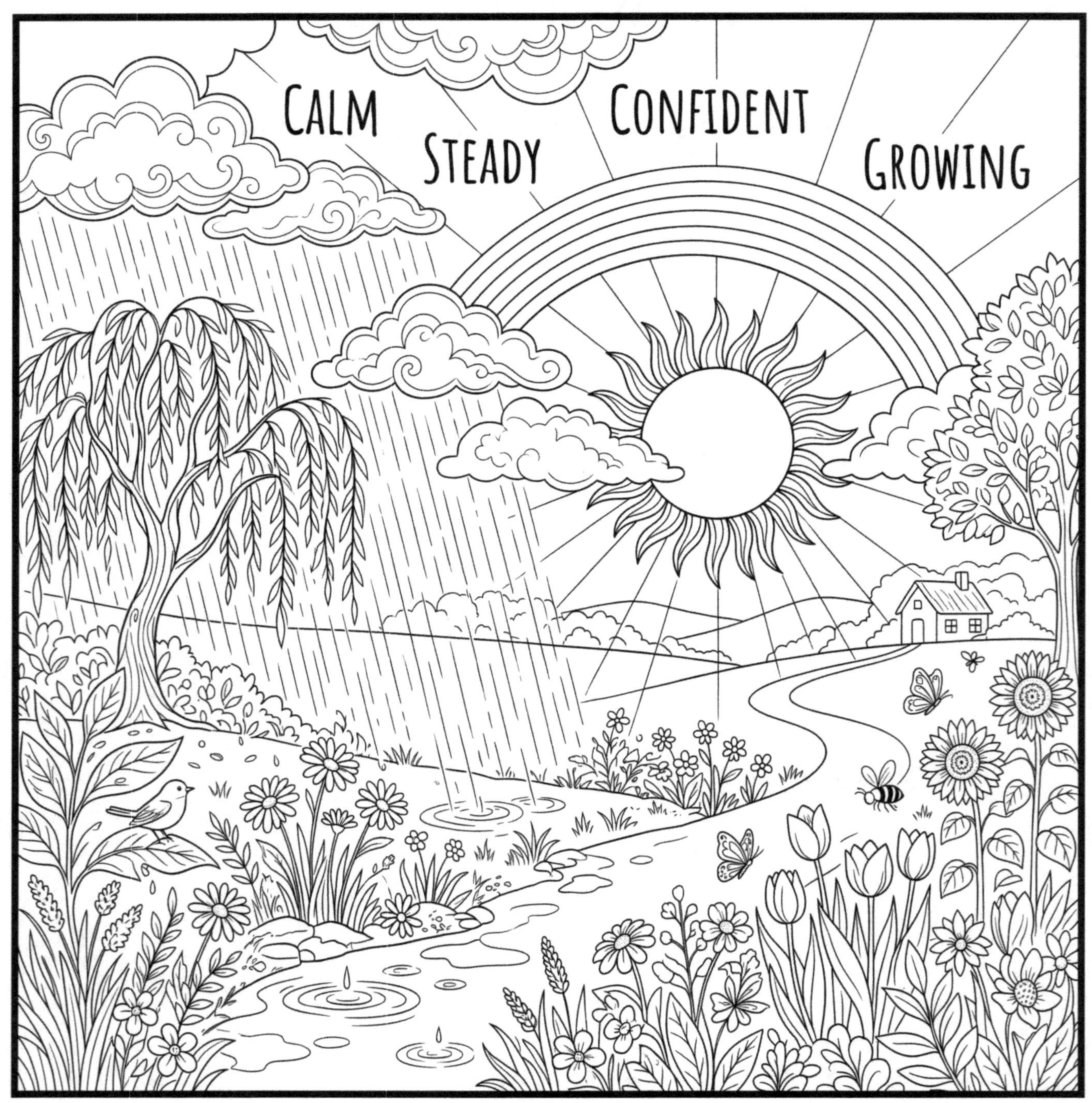

SECTION FOUR

Guard Your Peace

Protecting your peace is strength.

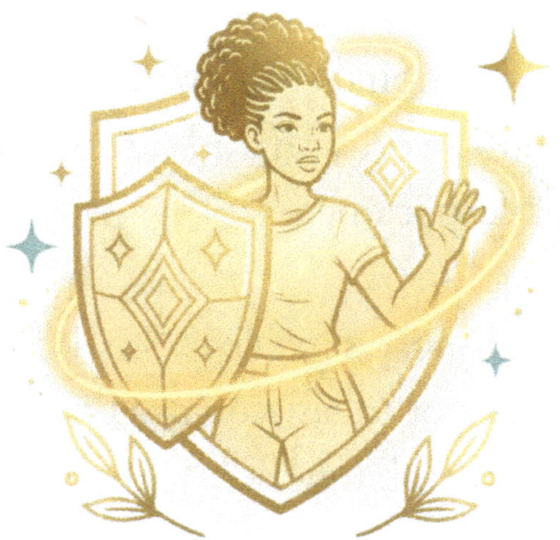

“Turn your wounds into wisdom.”
— Oprah Winfrey

Stress and Your Cycle

Your brain and body are deeply connected. You cannot have one without the other. Whenever you feel stressed, your body responds.

Stress hormones can influence your menstrual cycle. During stressful seasons, your period may arrive later than expected. You may notice stronger cramps. You may feel more irritable. You may feel more tired, even after resting. This does not mean something is wrong.

Your body is adjusting to hormonal shifts while also responding to your environment. Hormones guide growth and development, but they also influence mood, energy, and patience.

On some days, you may feel more sensitive. Small frustrations may feel larger than usual. That does not mean you are dramatic or difficult. It means your body is processing change.

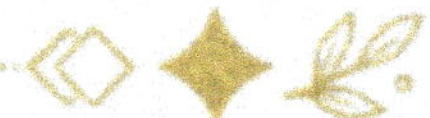

Learning to have patience with yourself during these moments is important. Extending patience to others is just as important. Awareness allows you to respond with maturity instead of reacting with frustration.

When you notice irritability or exhaustion, take a self time-out. A self time-out is not a punishment. It is a reset. It is a short pause to calm your nervous system. Step away from noise if possible and sit quietly for a few minutes.

Take slow breaths. Drink water. Stretch your body gently.

Healthy coping skills help your body settle. Deep breathing slows your heart rate. Drawing or coloring relaxes your thoughts. Reading shifts your focus. Writing helps you name your emotions instead of holding them inside. Proper rest and hydration support your body during hormonal shifts. Talking to someone you trust can release stress before it builds up.

Always guard your edges during stressful moments and choose calm over chaos.

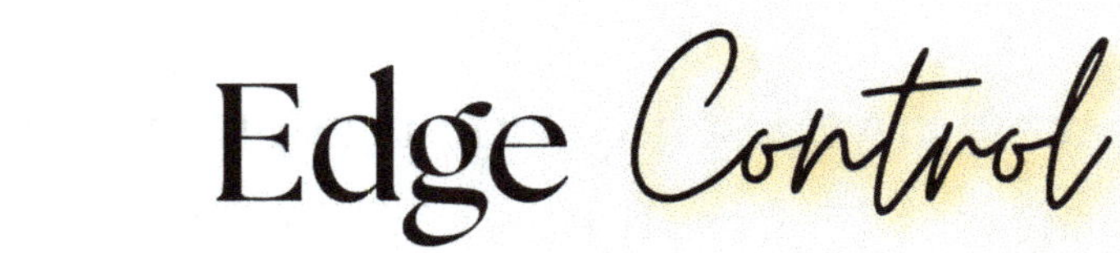

Edge Control

When emotions rise, pause before reacting.
Notice what your body needs.

Choose one healthy coping skill
and practice it intentionally.

Calm is a skill. The more you practice it,
the stronger it becomes.

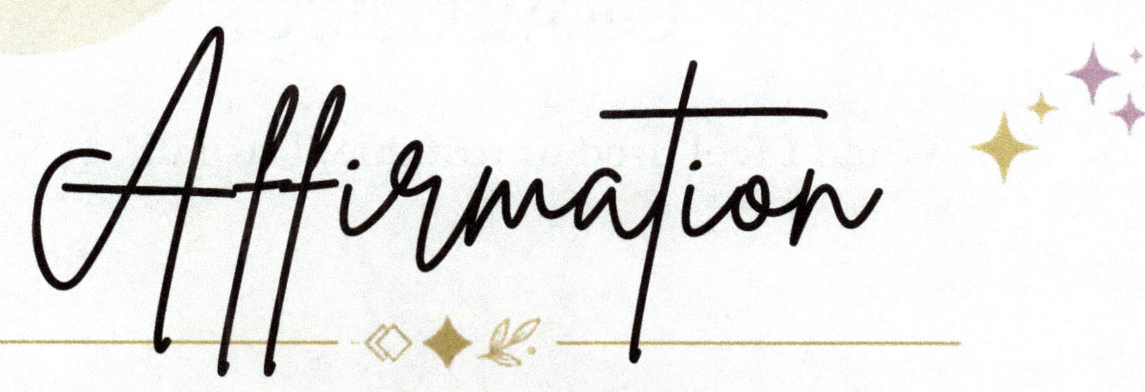

I can calm my body.

I am patient with myself as I grow.

I care for my mind, body, and soul.

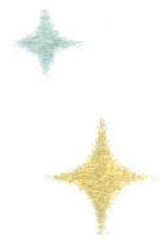

Glow Check

When I feel tired or irritable, I usually

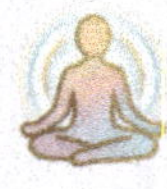

One coping skill I can try is

I show myself patience by

Breathe In Calm. Breathe Out Stress.

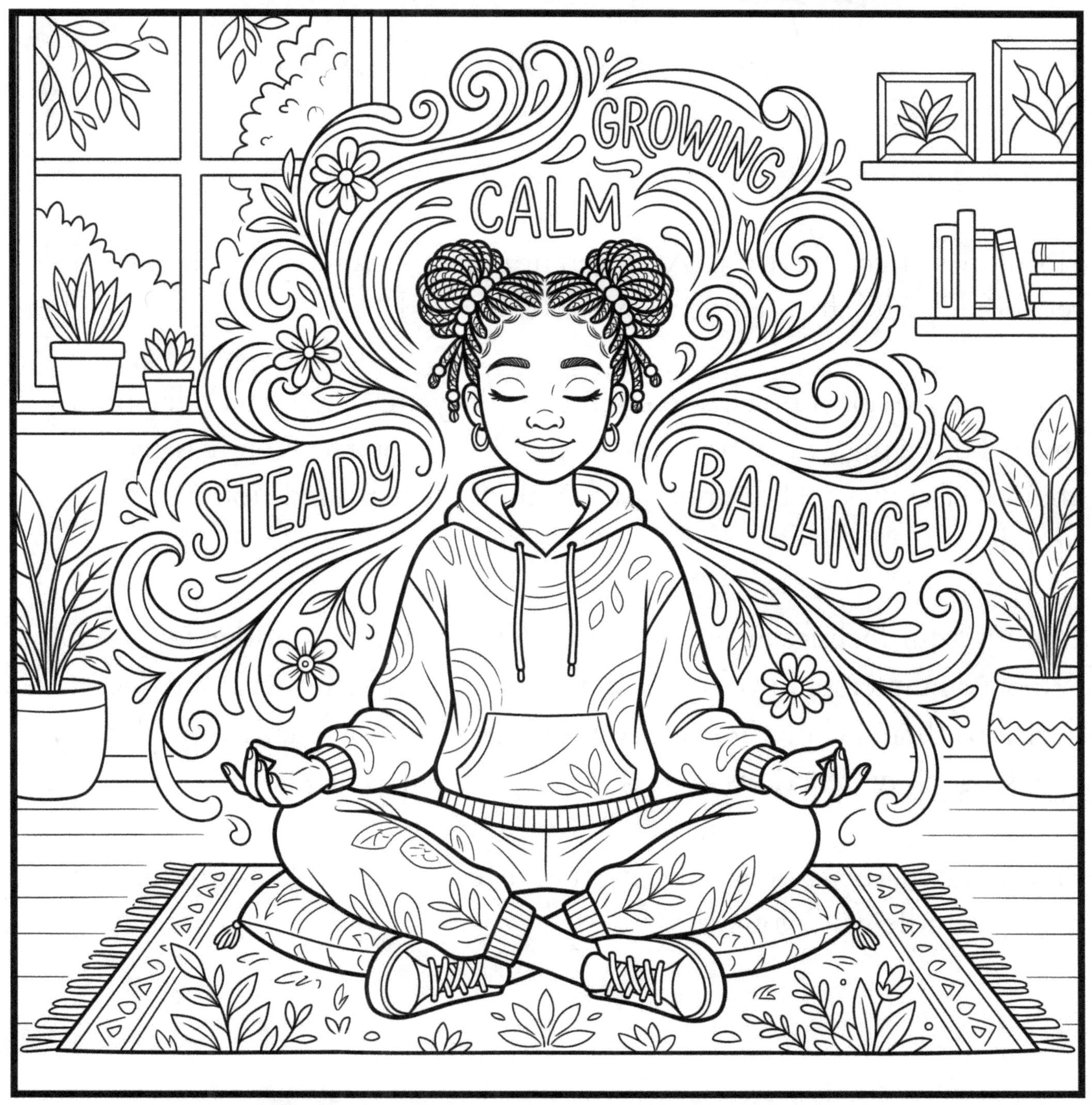

Let your breathing match your coloring.

Emotions and Clarity

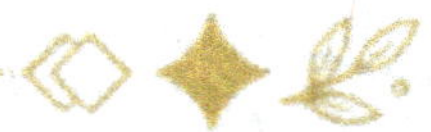

Hormones affect emotions. At different points in your cycle, you may feel reflective, joyful, focused, sensitive, or frustrated.

Emotions are not problems to eliminate. They are signals to understand. Instead of saying, "I feel bad," try naming what you feel. You may feel anxious. You may feel disappointed. You may feel excited. You may feel proud.

Naming your feelings gives you clarity. Clarity builds confidence. When you understand your emotions, you respond with wisdom. You make decisions thoughtfully. You speak with intention. You guard your glow by choosing steady reactions.

Emotional maturity does not mean never feeling upset. It means knowing how to handle what you feel.

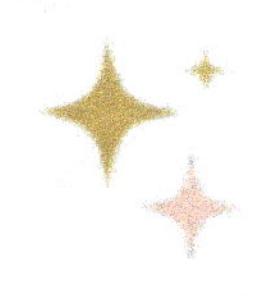

Edge *Control*

Before responding to a strong emotion, take one breath.

Ask yourself what you are feeling and what you need.

Awareness protects your peace.

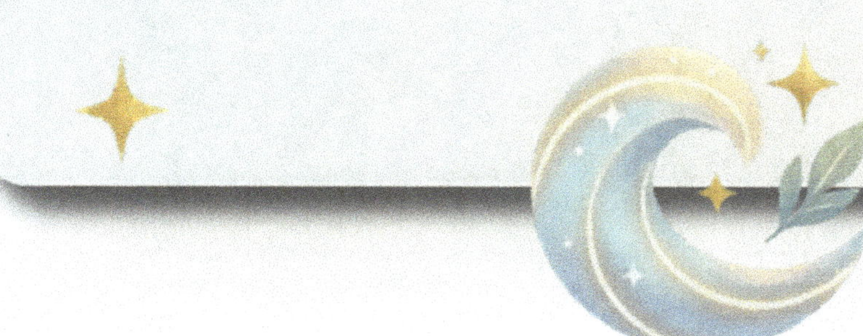

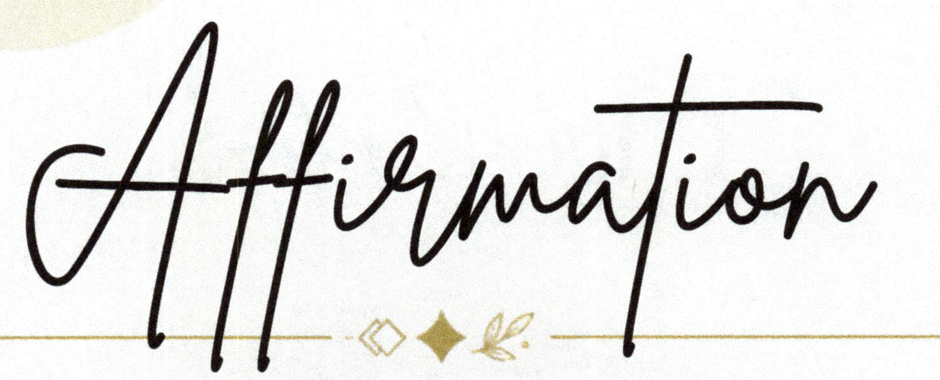

I understand my emotions.

I practice the pause.

I respond with wisdom and calm.

Glow Check

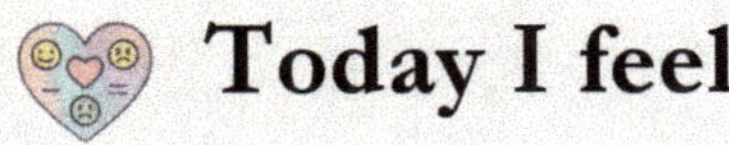

Today I feel

Naming my feelings helps me

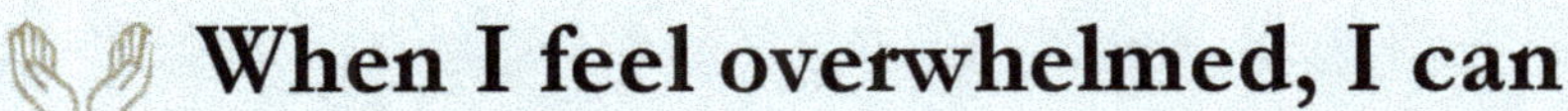

When I feel overwhelmed, I can

Understanding your emotions helps you guard your peace internally. Caring for your body daily helps you show that confidence externally.

Let us talk about handling your period with confidence and maturity.

SECTION FIVE

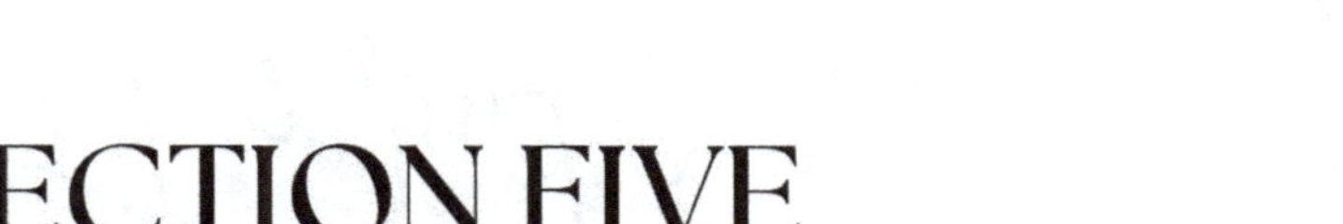

Handle it With Confidence

Preparation builds calm.
Calm builds confidence.

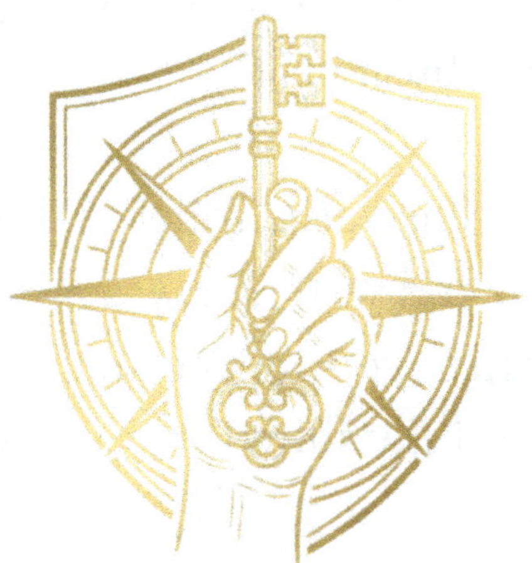

"I am deliberate and afraid of nothing."

— Audre Lorde

Managing your period is about responsibility and self-respect. When changing a pad, remove it carefully. Fold it inward so the used side is not visible. Wrap it in its original wrapper or tissue or even a plastic bag. Place it securely in the trash. Menstrual products should never be flushed.

Being clean and discreet is part of maturity. Discreet means handling your hygiene in a way that protects your privacy and keeps shared spaces comfortable for everyone. When you wrap products properly and dispose of them neatly, no one needs to know what you changed or when. In other words, **Your business is Your business.**

Before leaving the restroom, check the toilet seat and floor. Wash your hands thoroughly with soap and water. Always leave any space cleaner than you find it. These habits reflect confidence and responsibility, not shame. Caring for your body respectfully shows that you value yourself and the environment around you.

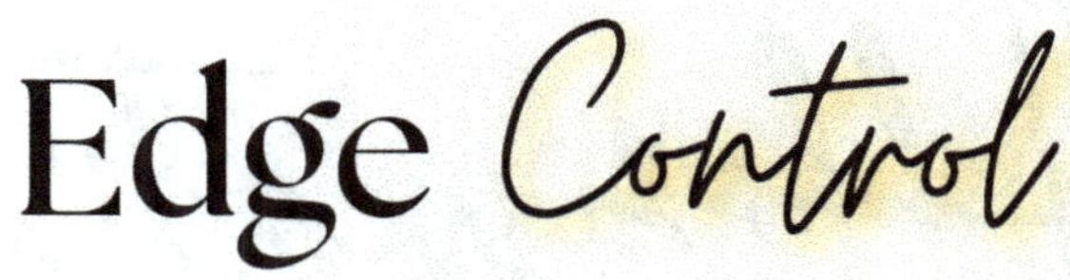

Edge *Control*

Small habits build strong confidence.

Handling your body with care strengthens your self-respect.

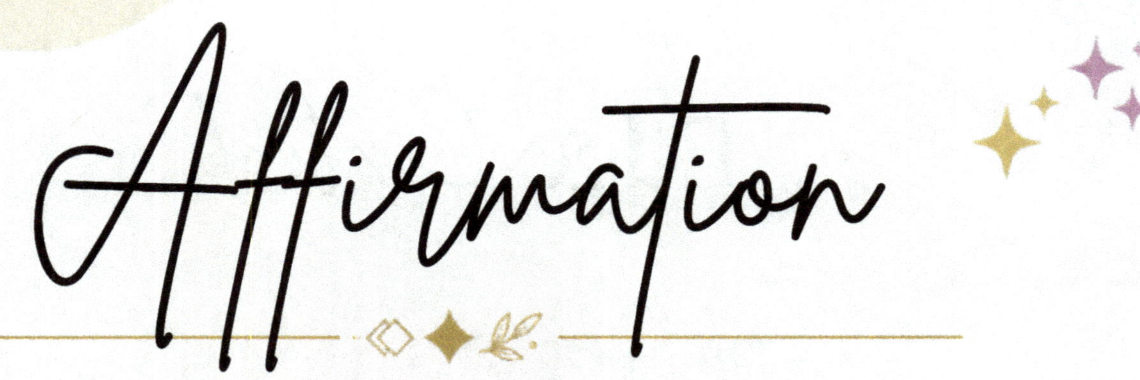

I handle my body with dignity

and responsibility.

Glow Check

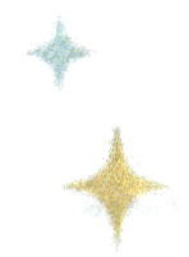

Today I feel

Naming my feelings helps me

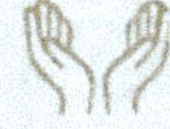

When I feel overwhelmed, I can

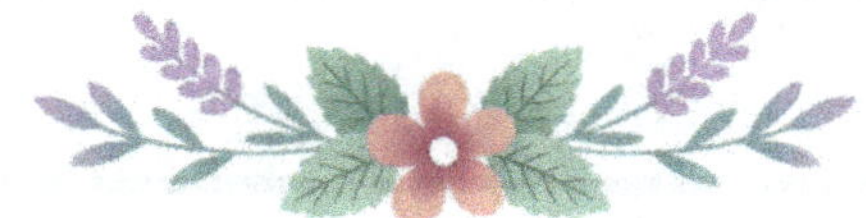

Design My Period Kit

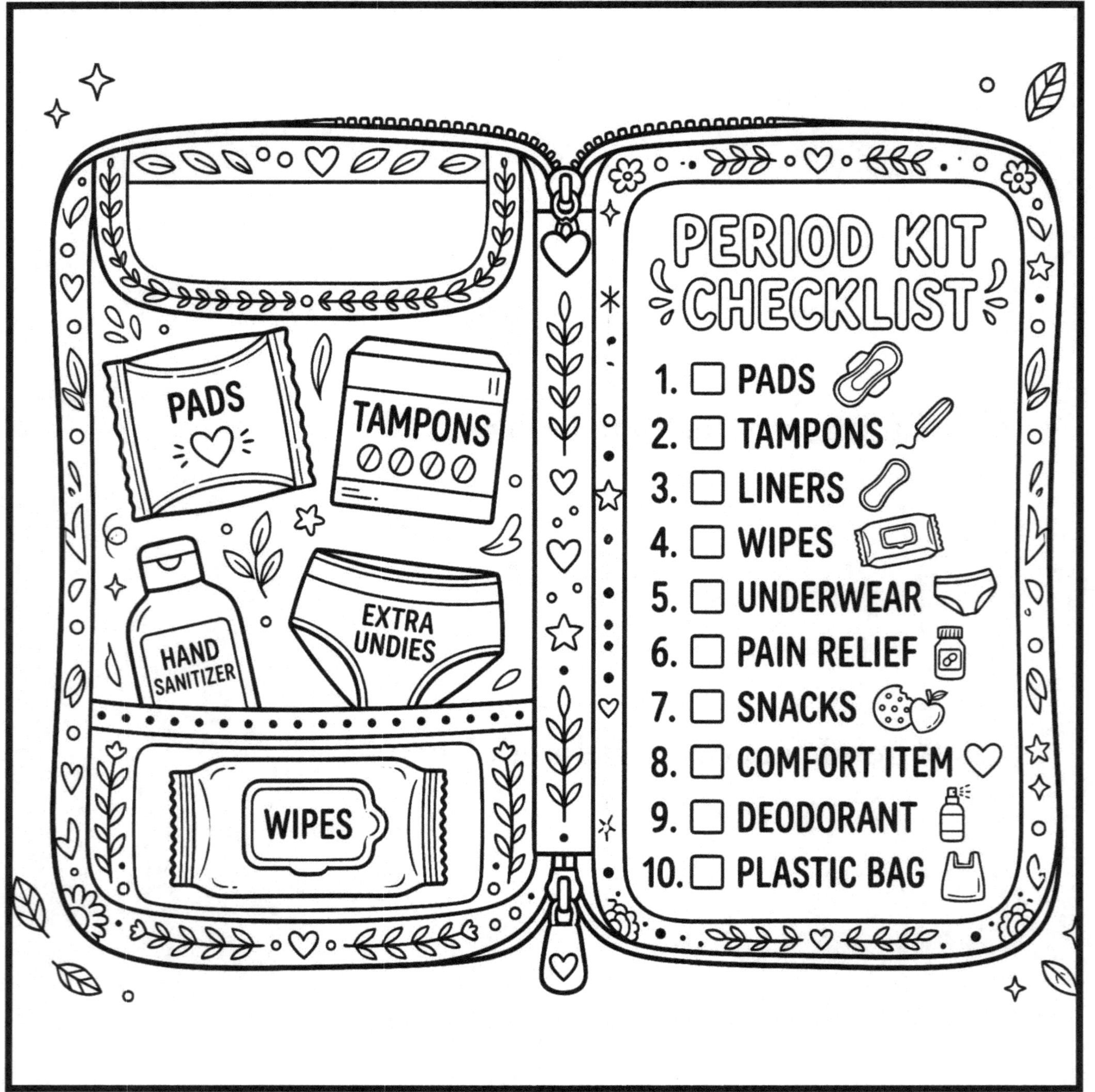

Prepared and Peaceful

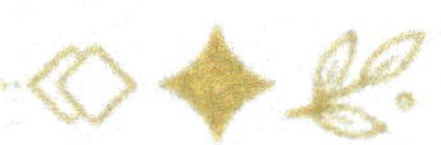

Creating a period pouch before you actually need it is one of the smartest ways to take care of yourself. It helps you feel ready instead of rushed, calm instead of confused. When your body begins to change, preparation gives you a sense of control and confidence.

A period pouch is a small bag or kit that you keep with you so you are prepared when your period starts or while you are on your cycle. It can be kept in your backpack, purse, locker, or school bag. Think of it as your personal care kit that helps you stay clean, comfortable, and confident throughout the day.

Your period pouch should include menstrual products such as pads, tampons (if you use them), or period underwear. It is also helpful to pack a pair of spare underwear in case of leaks. Adding wipes can help you freshen up when you are at school or away from home, and hand sanitizer is important for keeping your hands clean before and after changing your products.

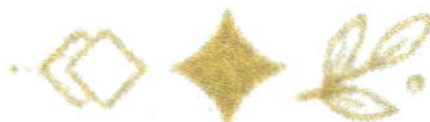

If you are active in sports, dance, or other activities, you may also want to include an extra pair of tights, shorts, or leggings for added security and comfort.

There are important reasons to create a period pouch. Periods do not always start at the exact same time every month, especially when your body is still growing and adjusting. Having a pouch ready helps you avoid feeling surprised or unprepared. It also reduces anxiety about leaks, stains, or not having supplies when you need them. Instead of worrying, you can stay focused on school, friendships, and the activities you enjoy.

Preparation creates calm and confidence. Learning how to be ready for your period is one of the first ways you can take care of your changing body with confidence. When you prepare, you protect your peace. You remove unnecessary stress and give yourself the ability to handle whatever your body does. You are telling yourself, "I am ready. I can take care of myself." Being prepared allows you to focus on what truly matters—learning, growing, laughing, and showing up as your full self with confidence.

Glow Check

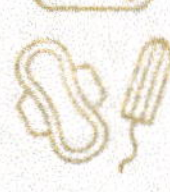

My period pouch will include

Being prepared helps me feel

I protect my peace by

SECTION SIX

Becoming

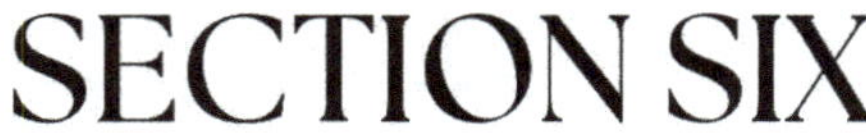

Growth is steady.

Becoming takes time.

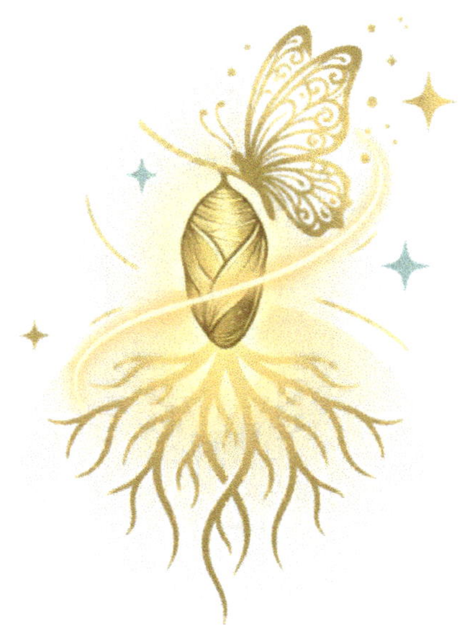

“Your story is what you have, what you will always have.”

— Michelle Obama

Becoming

Becoming means growing into yourself with intention. It is not about rushing toward adulthood. It is not about comparing your timeline to anyone else’s. It is about understanding who you are in each stage of life. Growth is not loud. It is steady.

Your menstrual cycle mirrors that process. Each month your body prepares. Each month it releases. Each month it renews. That rhythm reflects something deeper about you. You are always preparing for what is next. You are always releasing what no longer serves you. You are always renewing your strength.

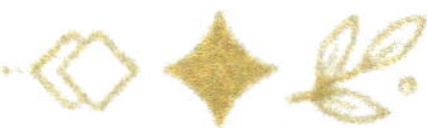

Becoming means recognizing your patterns without judgment. It means noticing what makes you feel strong and what makes you feel overwhelmed. It means honoring your body without apology. Some days you will feel confident. Other days you will feel uncertain. Both are part of growth.

You are not meant to shrink yourself to fit into a room. You are not meant to silence your voice to make others comfortable. You are meant to grow into your full presence with calm confidence. Your period is one part of your story. It does not define you, but it does teach you. It teaches you about rhythm. It teaches you about preparation. It teaches you about resilience.

Becoming is not about being perfect. It is about being aware.
When you guard your glow, you protect your peace. When you protect your peace, you create space to grow without fear.
You are becoming thoughtful.
You are becoming prepared.
You are becoming steady.
You are becoming strong.
That growth belongs to you.

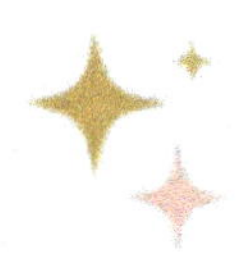

Edge *Control*

When you feel pressure to grow too fast, pause.

Remind yourself that growth unfolds at its own pace.

Protect your peace. Trust your process.

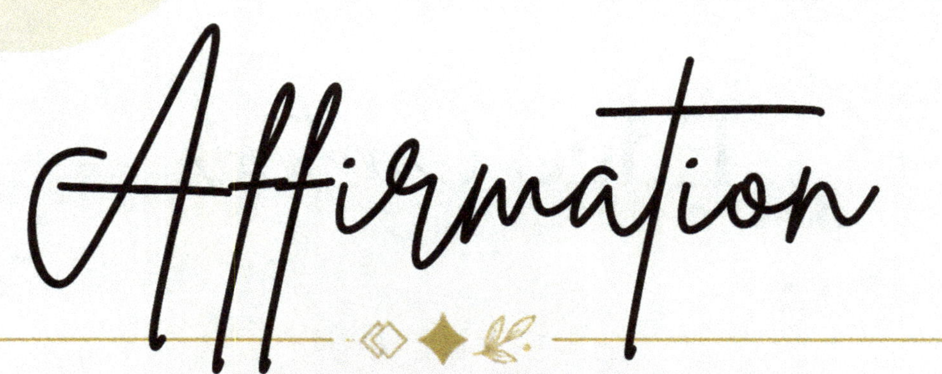

I am becoming confident, prepared,

and proud of who I am.

My growth is steady and intentional.

I trust my journey.

Glow Check

One way I have grown this year is

I feel most confident when

I can guard my glow by

Becoming Her

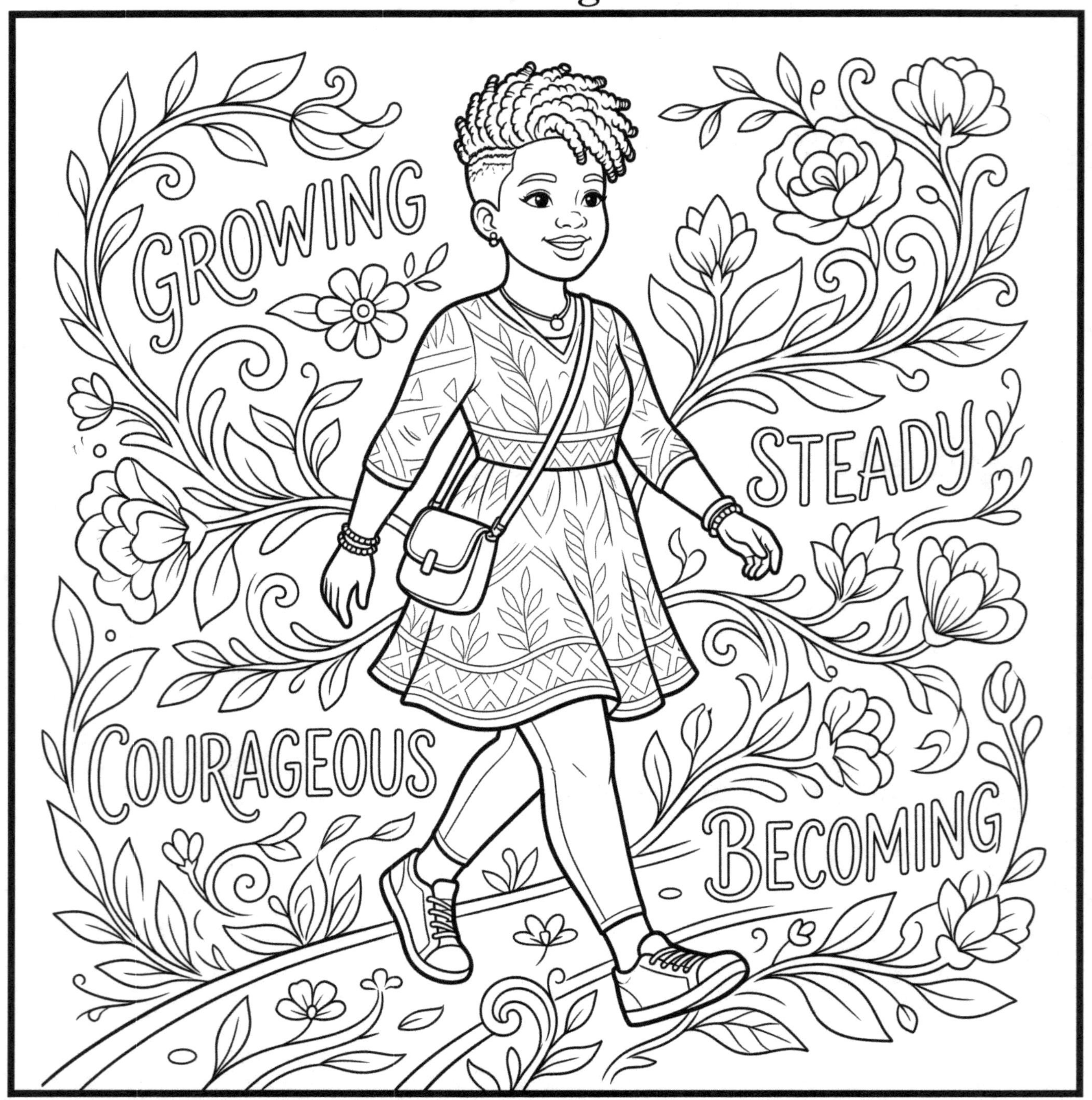

Growth belongs to you.

WORKBOOK SECTION

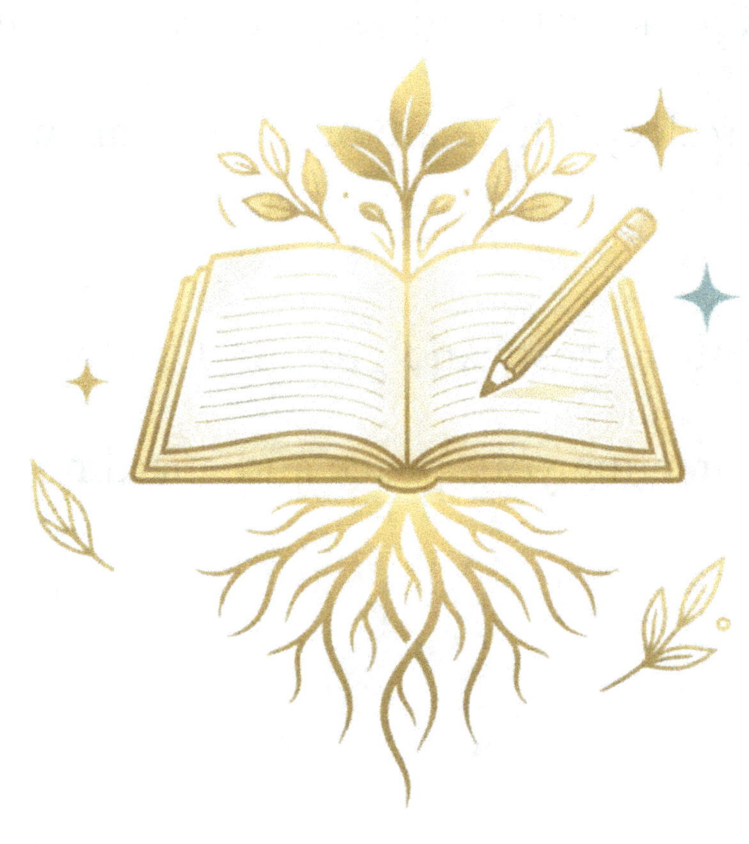

REFLECTION & PRACTICE

Learning about your body builds knowledge.

Writing about your experiences builds confidence.

This workbook section gives you space to think, plan, and reflect. There are no perfect answers.

There is only honesty and growth. Use these pages to practice protecting your peace and guarding your glow.

MY FIRST PERIOD PLAN

Planning reduces worry. Thinking ahead builds calm confidence. Use this page to write down what you will pack, who you will tell, and how you will care for yourself.

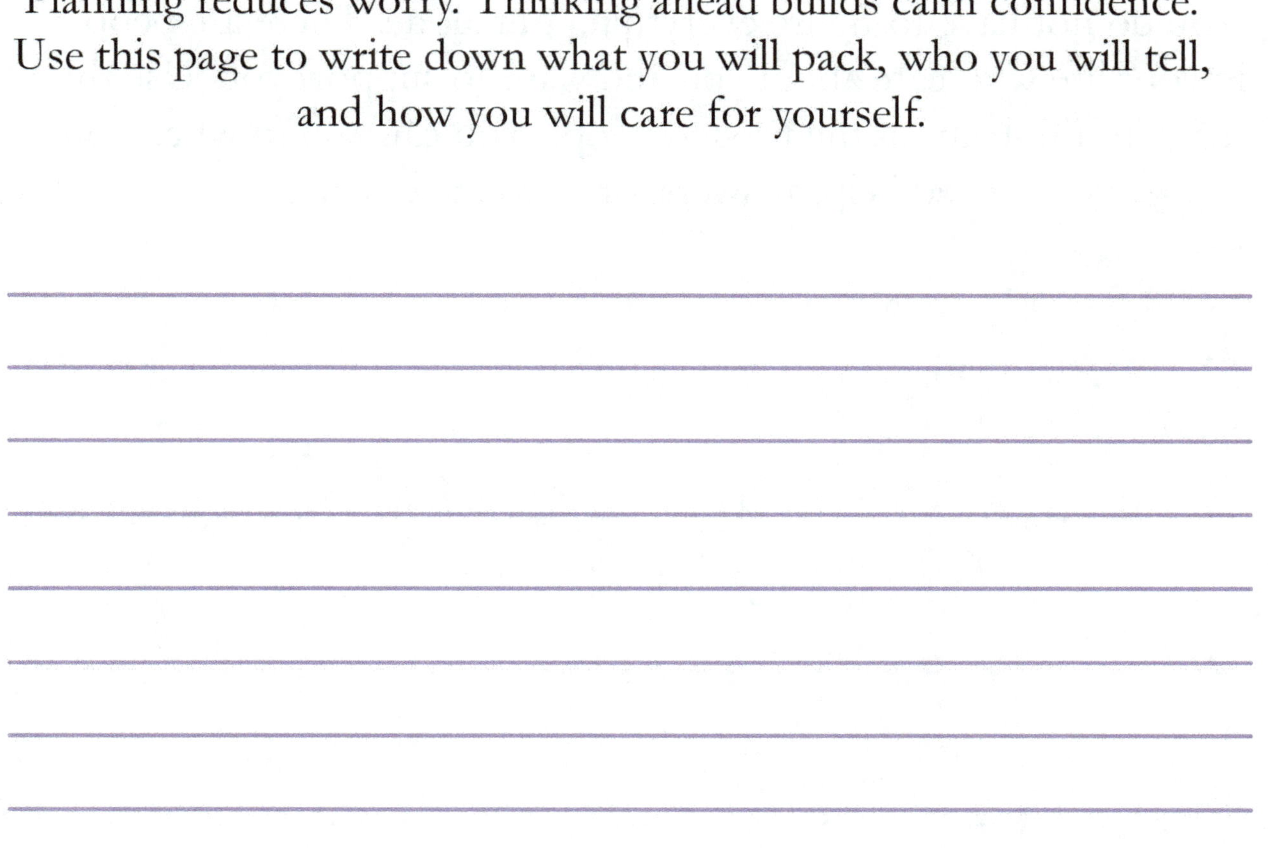

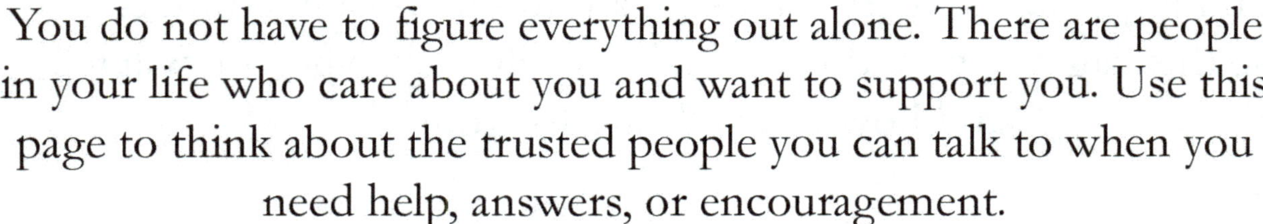

FIVE PEOPLE I CAN TALK TO

You do not have to figure everything out alone. There are people in your life who care about you and want to support you. Use this page to think about the trusted people you can talk to when you need help, answers, or encouragement.

1. ______________________________

2. ______________________________

3. ______________________________

4. ______________________________

5. ______________________________

SELF-CARE DURING MY CYCLE

Caring for your body is not selfish. It is one of the best ways to protect your peace and help yourself feel better. Use this page to think about the foods, activities, and habits that help you feel calm, rested, and strong during your cycle.

THINGS THAT HELP ME FEEL: CALM, RESTED, STRONG

Foods & Nutrition for my body

Activities and gentle movement

Routines and self-care habits

MONTHLY CYCLE TRACKER

Tracking your cycle helps you understand your body better.

DATE						
1	2	3	4	5	6	7
8	9	10	11	12	13	14
15	16	17	18	19	20	21
22	23	24	25	26	27	28
29	30	31				

MONTH:

YEAR:

MEDICATIONS:

PERIOD WAS

- ON TIME
- EARLY
- LATE
- HEAVY
- MEDIUM
- LIGHT

FEELING

- HAPPY
- SAD
- ANGRY
- ANNOYED
- TIRED
- SCARED

ANY SYMPTOMS?

- CRAMPS
- SORE BREAST
- HEADACHE
- FATIGUE
- ACNE
- CRAVINGS

CYCLE LENGTH

JAN	JUL
FEB	AUG
MAR	SEP
APR	OCT
MAY	NOV
JUN	DEC

NEXT PERIOD IS EXPECTED ON

DAY SINCE LAST PERIOD

PATTERN REFLECTION PAGE

Patterns help you understand what your body may need. You may notice certain feelings, cravings, or energy changes around the same time each month. Use this page to reflect on what you have noticed and what helps you feel your best.

Emotional/Mood Changes

Energy Levels

Cravings

____

____

____

____

____

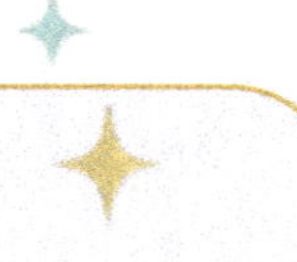

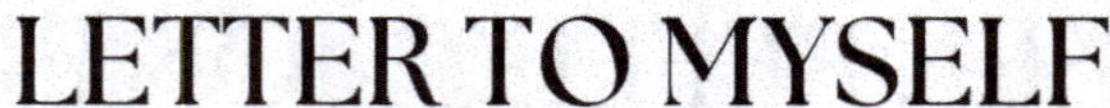

LETTER TO MYSELF

You are learning so much about yourself as you grow. Sometimes it helps to slow down and speak to yourself with kindness and encouragement. Use this page to write a letter reminding yourself of your strength, your growth, and everything you are becoming.

FINAL BLESSING

May you grow without shame.

May you move with grace in every season.

May you rest when your body asks for care.

May you listen when your heart asks for patience.

May you guard your glow with wisdom and confidence.

May you protect your peace without apology.

Becoming is not a race.

Becoming is a steady unfolding that belongs to you.

www.ingramcontent.com/pod-product-compliance
Lightning Source LLC
LaVergne TN
LVHW081420110826
845149LV00010B/1815

* 9 7 9 8 9 9 5 7 5 7 3 0 6 *